A Breast Cancer Journey to GREATER Joy!

Taking the fear and mystery out of a breast cancer diagnosis!

Joyce Fields

ISBN-13: 978-1499677980

Available at

amazon.com and other retailers
goodshortbooks.com

FOREWORD #1

It is my pleasure to write this foreword for Joyce Fields. Joyce has been on a breast cancer journey, not of her own choice, for the past several years. She is doing remarkably well and remains cancer free. Joyce has a wonderful attitude, great love and support from family and friends as well as outstanding support and treatment from extraordinary professionals, namely Dr. Stanley Tu (Internal Medicine), Dr. Dawn Hills (Surgery) and Dr. Helen Chen (Radiation Oncology). Joyce has taken charge of this cancer challenge and remains an inspiration to all of us. Her spirit shines through this wonderful memoir.

Mark V. McNamara, MD
Hematology/Oncology

<u>FOREWORD #2</u>

Mrs. Fields' memoir recounting her experience with cancer is an honest look at the trials and tribulations that cancer patients endure. Her battle with cancer has ended in success. She is doing very well. I am honored to have been part of the team of physicians that helped her through this tough part of her life.   It has been a pleasure getting to know Mrs. Fields through the years. She has a great outlook on life and has taught me a thing or two about courage and positive thinking. I look forward to our visits in the office and being greeted with a great big smile and hug.

Stanley S. Tu, MD
Internal Medicine

FOREWORD #3

I had the pleasure of caring for Joyce Fields during her radiation treatment in 2011. I recall her at that time being a woman with a uniquely positive attitude.

Joyce writes an extremely straightforward and easy-to-read book, with everything explained in lay terms. I believe that her personal recollection of the details of undergoing breast cancer treatment and the decision making involved offers great support to other patients because they are able to essentially relive her experience through reading this book.

Details regarding the emotions she went through, interactions with family members, scheduling appointments, reactions to big machines like radiation machines and PET/CT scanners are vividly recounted. Treatment involves visits to so many different physicians and undergoing so many tests.

Reading Joyce's book ahead of time would greatly prepare patients regarding what to expect. Early-stage breast cancer is generally a highly-curable disease. However, the word "cancer" is extremely stressful, and Joyce takes the mystery out of treatment of early-stage breast cancer.

Anyone anxious following a diagnosis of early-stage breast cancer (and who isn't?!) should read this book. It will greatly help them prepare for the road ahead.

Finally, having a positive attitude like Joyce's is actually immensely helpful in meeting the challenges of breast cancer treatment among other life's challenges.

Helen Chen, MD
Radiation Oncology

FOREWORD #4

I have the privilege of writing a foreword for this account of one woman's journey through the diagnosis and treatment of breast cancer.

I was fortunate to have been the breast surgeon for Joyce Fields. Her positive attitude during and after surgery provided the optimum scenario for healing of both body and spirit.

Through this book she provides a path of hope for women beginning a similar, unwelcome journey.

I encourage them to find inspiration and hope through her example.

Dawn M. Hills, M.D.

INTRODUCTION

This memoir was written as a source of inspiration for anyone who has been diagnosed with breast cancer, especially with Stage 2 invasive ductal carcinoma and hormone receptive, and chose (or will choose) to have a lumpectomy and radiation, as I did. Chances are that you'll have to go through what I went through, as described in this chronicle of my breast cancer journey.

It includes my daily experiences, information that I found to be useful, foods and supplements that can help you improve your health, and the acknowledgement of how important it is to have loved ones share in the experience.

I believe in God, but whatever you call your "Higher Power," faith plays a crucial role in eliminating fear.

It is my sincere prayer that something shared within this account of what could have been a despairing passage in my life, will provide someone with the encouragement, advice, inspiration, courage, and support they need to transform their diagnosis into **their** positive experience!

BEGINNING THE JOURNEY

I retired in May 2010 at the age of 66.

In mid May 2011, I was scheduled for and had a mammogram.

In late May 2011, my doctor's office informed me that my mammogram was abnormal, and that the doctor wanted me to take another one.

The second one showed a small "nodule" in my right breast.

In June 2011, I was diagnosed with breast cancer.

BACKGROUND

About 30 years ago, I felt a lump in my left breast.

I never considered myself to be a worrier, but I must have been worried about it; my spirit was more upset than I wanted to believe it was, because. . .

One night, I was in that "twilight sleep," where you're either just falling off to sleep or just about to wake up. I don't know which it was.

I heard this voice—loud and clear. It was the voice of a man. It slowly and deliberately said, "YOU. DO. NOT. HAVE. BREAST. CANCER."

It sounded like it came from the foot of the bed. I was on my back, so I raised my head to see if someone or something was there. I saw no one and nothing. It must have been God or one of His angels! I didn't wake my husband (everybody calls him "Pap") because I was not apprehensive at all.

I laid back down, with the most profound sense of peace that I've ever experienced.

Soon thereafter, my sisters, Nita and Ava, went with me on my doctor's visit. We held hands as the doctor announced that **THE LUMP WAS GONE**! He said that it probably was a cyst that drained itself. Or, I thought, *it could have been a miracle!*

Fast forward to June 2011. . .

ONWARD AND UPWARD

During my visit to my Primary Care Physician, Dr. Stanley Tu of Pasadena, California, in June 2011, when he told me that the mammogram showed a small "nodule" in my right breast, I told him about my message from God or one of His angels some thirty years prior.

We both smiled when I told him that the messenger didn't say I would NEVER have breast cancer. I guess I wanted to believe it to be life-long.

Oh, well, back to reality.

My next step was to have a needle core biopsy. That made me a bit nervous, but I figured that others had gone through it and survived—so would I! Everything connected to a breast cancer diagnosis was a mystery to me. I didn't have a clue as to what was in store. But I was not scared. I just wanted it GONE!

June 23 was "biopsy day." Pap went with me. Thank goodness! It was a breeze! Really!! The worst part was the injection to deaden the breast, and it wasn't as bad as the injection to deaden your gums for a root canal or a tooth extraction.

I felt nothing during the actual biopsy procedure. I was relaxed and comfortable. Using a computer screen, the doctor guided the instrument to the nodule and cut three snippets. He told me when to expect to hear the "click" as the instrument made the cut. I heard it, but didn't feel it. The entire procedure took less than 30 minutes.

The nurse placed an ice pack over the biopsy site (a little bigger than a needle prick mark) and gave me instructions on how to keep my breast cold for the next several hours, which helps with swelling, pain, and discomfort. The instructions said to use frozen green peas. Yep, green peas! We had to stop and buy a couple of bags of frozen green peas. They're very pliable and work wonders as an ice pack. I divided the bag into smaller bags. And my bra worked wonders in keeping it in place. That did the job—I had absolutely no swelling, pain, or discomfort from the biopsy!

The Huntington-Hill Breast Center in Pasadena, California, is a fantastic, state-of-the-art, beautiful facility. The staff treats patients with tremendous professionalism, courtesy, kindness, and sensitivity. Kudos to all of them!

The next day—on June 24—the doctor called to tell me that they found cancer cells in the biopsy specimen. Awww, crap!

I didn't cry. I was in a state of shock, realizing that **I HAD BREAST CANCER!!** I didn't feel like I had breast cancer. I felt wonderful, great, fantastic!! I had been saying for 30 years that I didn't feel any differently than I felt when I was 30 years old!! No aches. No pains. No medications. But to learn that I had breast cancer. . .WOW!! I just wanted it **OUT**!!

I was instructed to make an appointment to see Dr. Tu, which I did.

On my next visit to Dr. Tu, he gave me several referrals from which I could choose the doctors I would see. There were two surgeons (I think I was divinely guided to choose Dr. Dawn Hills); one radiology oncologist, Dr. Helen Chen; and one medical oncologist, Dr. Mark McNamara, all of Pasadena, and all within three or four miles of each other. That's VERY important in California because getting from Point A to Point B can be a real traffic nightmare!

Back in April—before I knew there was a lump in my breast—I had already bought my ticket to Detroit, where I make a yearly visit to see my family. My two sisters (Nita and Ava) and three of my four brothers (George, Cordell, and Kenny) still live there—the place where we were born and raised, and where I lived until 2003. My fourth brother (Reggie) lives in Springfield, Massachusetts. (Sadly, George passed away on April 28, 2013--from lung cancer.)

I look forward to seeing my siblings, as well as grandkids, nieces, nephews, and a bunch of other relatives and friends. This trip was scheduled for July 2 to July 11, so I wanted to make my doctor's appointment AFTER I returned from Detroit. And I wanted to know if that would be okay.

Dr. Tu thought that would be fine, but he wanted me to consult with Dr. Hills.

I called Dr. Hills' assistant, Rebecca, and asked her to ask Dr. Hills if I could delay seeing her until after July 11. My appointment was scheduled for July 15. Yaaay!!

I very objectively calculated how and when I was going to tell my siblings and others about my breast cancer diagnosis. I did not want a "doom and gloom" overtone to my trip.

For ten whole days, I had an absolutely wonderful time in Detroit!

My flight back to LAX was to depart on July 11 at 10:15 p.m. About 30 minutes before leaving the house, heading to Detroit Metro Airport, I gathered all the females in an upstairs room and told them the good and bad news. The good news: early detection and a small lump; the bad news: it was cancerous.

Their faces were all glum, but brightened when I told them that I was feeling fine (hadn't I showed them that during the ten days?), and I wasn't sad or worried. It's in God's hands. I just wanted it **out of me**.

They had a few questions, followed by hugs and smiles. Then, I went downstairs and told the guys. They saw how I was handling it, so they handled it well, too.

I have a GREAT family!!

Hugs and kisses all around, then it was time to leave for the airport.

CALIFORNIA, HERE I COME!

I was ready to see Dr. Hills on July 15! Pap went with me, as usual. He was very supportive. (He has since told me that he was terrified!)

On July 15, I'm sitting in the examining room, waiting for Dr. Hills to enter. I'm very pleased with how calm I seem to be.

The technician knocks and enters the room to take my vitals. Height is 5' 2", weight is (I ain't tellin'), temperature is normal, and blood pressure is.........116/58! I **AM** calm!!

I have to take off my top and put on that paper jacket—open in the front.

Dr. Hills knocks and enters the room. She's blonde, tall, and slender, and very sharply dressed. I don't remember our initial conversation, but she performs a thorough breast exam, tells me to get dressed and that she'll wait for me outside the door, and we'll go to another room to talk.

Pap joins us. In the consultation room, she draws a picture of a breast—a front view and a side view.

I have the most common form of breast cancer—invasive ductal carcinoma. She draws milk ducts in the picture and explains that the cancer started in a duct and then burst out of it; hence, the "invasive" part. I understand. I just want it **out**.

She explains more medical stuff about lymph nodes, sentinel nodes, etc. She wants me to get an MRI so she can have a three-dimensional view of the lump.

I really like Dr. Hills! Good vibes! She explains thoroughly, answers all of our questions, and makes sure that we understand. And she has a great sense of humor!

A few days later, I had the MRI. The results showed a "suspicious" lymph node under my right arm. Another biopsy is necessary. I prayed that it was benign. My prayer was answered. It was just fatty tissue. I said, "Thank you, God!!"

Surgery (a lumpectomy) is scheduled for Monday, August 15.

Dr. Hills has ordered me to be on a "Club Med Vacation." So, for three weeks, I will do no cooking, cleaning, or laundry! That's gonna be very strange, but a girl's gotta do what a girl's gotta do! Or rather, a girl's gotta NOT do what a girl's gotta NOT do!

But, she explicitly told me that I <u>CAN</u> be on the computer. Woo hoo!!

MONDAY, AUGUST 15. SURGERY DAY! WOO HOO!!

Pap and I arrive at the Breast Center at 7:30 a.m.

I never thought I'd be happy to have surgery, but, when this is over, the cancerous tumor will be out of me! I'm happy, but calm. My blood pressure is 123/53.

They get my breast ready. A thorough swabbing, followed by two injections. One inserts a wire that comes out the side of my breast. The other inserts dye. Then I'm accompanied to the mammography room for a "gentle" mammogram. All of this will help guide Dr. Hills to the tumor.

They wheel me to the hospital. The nurse gets my IV set up. Dr. Parenti, the anesthesiologist (she's married to my Medical Oncologist, Dr. McNamara), comes in and asks me a lot of questions. She's funny. I like her, too.

That's all I remember until after surgery and recovery, when I'm being wheeled to my room. In addition to the lumpectomy, Dr. Hills removed seven lymph nodes (only one was cancerous). She had to insert a drainage tube in me, so I have to stay overnight. Pap stays with me, and that makes it better!

Tuesday morning Dr. Hills visits me. Everything went very well! Yaaay! She'll get the <u>official</u> results on Wednesday or Thursday and call me then. Hugs all around; then, she released me from the hospital.

I FEEL **REALLY** GOOD—emotionally, spiritually, and physically!

And I've never stopped praying!

The day after the surgery, Tuesday, August 16, I was back at home, feeling GREAT!! Virtually **no** pain! And soooo very glad that the tumor had been cut out of my breast!

I thank God all day, every day, but I was **REALLY** thanking Him on Tuesday!! So was everyone who loves and cares about me!

Later that evening, I was sitting in my Lazy Boy, just relaxing with my family (Pap; our son, Mkonto; Konto's girlfriend, Kortnie, and his two daughters, Mekkah [12] and Medina [16 months]). All of a sudden, the doorbell rings. Pap answers it. Walking through the front door is my sister, Nita—all the way from Detroit!! (So as not to cause any suspicion on my part, our family friend, John, picked her up from the airport.) What a shock!! I was totally surprised!! (She bought her ticket on July 12, the day after I announced to family and friends that I had been diagnosed with breast cancer and was scheduled to have surgery on August 15.) **WHAT A SISTER!!**

MY "CLUB MED" VACATION!

These days after surgery have been absolutely wonderful! Pap, Nita, and Mekkah are not allowing me to do anything around the house, which is weird for me, but that's what I need right now. A "Club Med" vacation!

Dr. Hills said that I could go walking, read, and work on the computer. So, I've walked (six blocks, roundtrip) to the "corner" store twice, gone to the grocery store twice, and gone to the mall once, I'm always reading something, and I work on the computer every day. For the trips to the grocery store and the mall, I was a passenger (one of my "do nots" is driving).

On Monday, August 22, Mekkah cooked dinner: chicken and corn soup. She got the recipe off the Internet and did an excellent job! It was DELICIOUS!! Mekkah wants to be a chef. She wants to go to Le Cordon Blue Culinary School in Paris, France! She's already checked out the airfare from LAX!

Since she wants to be a chef, Mekkah is thoroughly enjoying preparing meals for us. She makes my most basic requests look beautiful.

Good support makes for a better, faster recovery, and my immediate support team—Pap,

Nita, and Mekkah—are really greasing the skids for me!! My extended support team—other family members and friends—are supporting me via visits, phone calls, e-mails, and social media.

Friday, August 26, was another "good news" day for me! I had a follow-up appointment with Dr. Hills.

When she came into the exam room, her first two, excited words were "Good news!" I kind of went into another zone from there. A very **happy** zone!!

I don't remember EXACTLY what she said after that, but THE cancer (not MY cancer—I have never claimed it!) is not very aggressive, and it is like its parent, meaning the cells in the tumor were the same as the cells in the duct from which it started. And that's a good thing! (It's hard to explain, but I think I got all of that right.)

In a week or so, I'll have my first meeting with my Medical Oncologist, Dr. Mark McNamara, who will assess all my results and advise and guide me on the medical part of the path ahead of me, further unraveling mysteries associated with the diagnosis.

NITA GOES BACK TO DETROIT

On Sunday, August 28, I'm a little sad because we took Nita to LAX for her morning flight back home to Detroit. Twelve days of talking, going, teaching Mekkah, watching movies, cooking, eating, watching the news, and sharing love and laughter. I am so very glad and thankful that she was here. I got a little misty on the ride back from LAX, but I know that she has to return to her life. She didn't even take a vacation day for Monday! Back to her job as an Executive Assistant.

We talk on the phone often, and she and our sister, Ava, will continue to be with me in this chapter of my life. Having Nita and Ava as sisters is truly wonderful!

KEEP ON BLOGGIN'

For my Saturday, August 27, post, I mentioned that "teaching Mekkah" was part of our routine. I'm always in "teaching mode" with her, but having Nita here—while I recovered from surgery—provided extra lessons and living examples of love, compassion, cooperation, selflessness, kindness, order and organization— all the good things that money cannot buy.

After reading that post, Mekkah submitted a comment, saying that she **was** learning "stuff."

I was curious to know what that "stuff" was. Here's some of what she said she learned:

- How to peel potatoes with a knife, instead of a potato peeler (I don't own and have never used a potato peeler).
- Love for family. She watched the way Nita and I interacted, and she liked the vibes between us. (She said she really couldn't explain. It was just a real good feeling.) Like me, Mekkah is a "big sister."
- Spelling tricks. I taught her my secret for knowing the difference between desert and dessert—if you're spelling "dessert," as in something sweet, think "**s**trawberry **s**hortcake" and use double "s." And I

taught her that "nieces" like "pieces" of "pie." It's "i" before "e" in all three cases. (But she should still remember the "i before e" rhyme.)

- How to make, bake, and slice a turkey loaf. I walked her through the entire process, and she did a fabulous job! It was delicious! Leftovers!
- How to thoroughly clean a kitchen. Move things; don't just wipe around them! Don't leave dirty pots and pans on the stove!
- Honesty pays and makes you feel and look good. She thought she was finished with the kitchen, but there were a few potatoes left in the skillet, and she left them there—on the stove. When I saw them, I asked her why she left them there. Her response was, "I didn't know what you wanted me to do with them." The only problem with that answer is that **SHE DIDN'T ASK ME!** I let her know that that was totally unacceptable and it made her look shady.

She said she understood. We'll see.

KORTNIE AND MEKKAH TAKE OVER

Well, the last "My Breast Cancer Journey" post was on August 29, the day after we took Nita to LAX for her return trip to Detroit. It was sooooo good having her with me. As well as being wonderful company for Mekkah and me (the three of us had a lot of fun!), she drove my car to take me to doctor visits, the grocery store— wherever I needed or wanted to go. And she and Mekkah did all my cooking and housework. (I was on doctor's orders **not** to drive, cook, or do housework.)

Here's some of what happened since August 29:

- After Nita left, Kortnie volunteered to be my driver and helper, along with Mekkah. What an angel! She would spend the night on the night before my doctor visits and also take me on any errands that I had to run. And she would bring my 17- month-old, delightful granddaughter, Medina, with her! So, Mekkah, Kortnie, Medina, and I had a really good time— cooking, eating, watching movies, playing cards. I was thrilled to have both my son's daughters AND his girlfriend with me!

Pap joined in the eating and playing cards, but he didn't too much like our choices in movies, and there's only so much estrogen he can take in one dose. LOL! So, on some days, he would seek out testosterone, knowing that I was doing very well and in good hands.

- At the end of my surgery on August 15, Dr. Hills inserted a drain in me to collect the lymph fluid that flowed as a result of having seven lymph nodes removed.

The drain did not cause any pain or discomfort, but had to be emptied, and the contents measured, three times each day. This ingenious contraption had a tube that was about 10 inches long by 1/8 inch wide, connected to a small vacuum bulb that gently sucked out the lymph fluid. It fit comfortably inside my bra.

Pap was very diligent about helping me to do this. (This was not as gory as it may sound! It was exciting to watch the fluid level go down and to watch the odorless fluid get clearer and clearer.) The measurement started out at 40cc total for the day on August 16, went as high as 87cc total for the day on August 26. The goal was to have less than a total of 30cc on **two** consecutive days! That happened on

September 2 (27cc) and September 3 (22cc)—
yippeee!!! It dwindled down to 7cc on
September 5, but, unfortunately, it was a
weekend, so I had to wait for my appointment
on Tuesday, September 6 (my late father's
birthday!).

On September 6, Dr. Hills removed the
bandages and the drain. It was a painless
procedure—just a very slight pinch when she
snipped the one stitch that held the drainage
tube in place. She applied a small bandage over
the opening where the drainage tube had been
and told me to come back on September 9 (my
late maternal grandmother's birthday!).

My family members' birthdays have always been
good omens for me. I started my very first job
on my mother's birthday, April 9 (1962)!

LIBERATION!!

I went back to see Dr. Hills on September 9.

She removed the small bandage that covered the opening where the drainage tube had been, examined the incision where she removed the tumor and the incision where she removed the lymph nodes. She told me that I was healing— her word was, "perfectly." Yaaay!!

Naturally, scar tissue had formed on both incisions, but I didn't feel any tightness on my breast. I could, however, feel the tightness on the lymph node incision (that was right at the base of my right armpit)—I could not lift my arm straight up and stretch it out completely without some discomfort.

She showed me the exercise that I would have to do five times every morning and five times every night for five to six weeks: Stand where the wall creates a right angle. Place both heels against the wall, back straight, shoulders on the wall. Raise both arms to shoulder height, with my right hand (palm flat) on the opposite wall. Walk my fingers (Pap laughs and says my fingers are "tip-toeing") up the wall. Go as far as possible, then step in a bit and continue the finger walk. When I'm about 10 or 12 inches from the wall, slide my hip in to rest on the wall, arm still extended, and fingers still walking as far as possible, touching my ear to my shoulder.

I did two in her office, so she could be sure I was doing them correctly. When I finished those two, I could already feel tremendous improvement in the tightness.

(I can now lift my arm straight up and stretch it completely out with no discomfort whatsoever! I'm only five feet, two inches tall, but, by the end of these five to six weeks of stretching, my fingers may be tip-toeing ON THE CEILING!)

Then Dr. Hills gave me the best news I've had since the surgery and the removal of the drainage tube. She told me I could start back to driving my car the next day!! Hallelujah!!!

The surgery phase is now complete. I don't have another appointment with her until December 7!

The next phase is consultation appointments with my Radiation Oncologist, Dr. Helen Chen, and my Medical Oncologist, Dr. Mark McNamara.

DRS. McNAMARA AND CHEN

On September 13, I had my consultation visits with my Medical Oncologist, Dr. Mark McNamara (Dr. Mac), and my Radiation Oncologist, Dr. Helen Chen.

It was logistically convenient because they're about a five-minute drive apart.

My diagnosis: Stage 2 breast cancer that is not very aggressive and is hormone receptive. Dr. Mac said that my outlook is "very, very good." Another blessing!

He explained the benefits of chemotherapy and Tamoxifen.

If I chose to do it, chemotherapy would consist of four sessions, which would increase my odds for a cure by 4% (1% per session). I think those odds are way too low, so I chose NOT to do chemotherapy. Dr. Mac said that, for me, it is "reasonable not to take chemo." And "the overall cure rate is still high."

This cancer being "hormone receptive" means that it is feeding off hormones. The Tamoxifen will decrease (but not stop) my hormone output, blocking the cancer's ability to feed, and the cells will die. I will take this pill twice a day, every day, for five years. Dr. Mac said that "Tamoxifen is more beneficial than chemo." That made me even more comfortable with my decision. Plus, Tamoxifen has been around for a long time. I know several breast cancer survivors who took it more than 10 or 20 years ago.

Additionally, Dr. Mac said that, for all his Stage 2 breast cancer patients, he recommends a whole-body PET scan to see if cancer cells are in other parts of the body. I will be scheduling an appointment for a PET scan.

Dr. Mac also said, "Surgery + radiation = mastectomy." I already had the surgery and was ready for my radiation consultation appointment with Dr. Chen.

At this point, I've had two sessions with Dr. Chen. At the first appointment, her nurse documented my health history and took my vitals; then Dr. Chen explained how radiation works. (The tumor has been surgically removed. The radiation will kill any remaining cancer cells in my breast.) The radiation is targeted to a specific area. My thyroid and heart will not receive any radiation. I was told that I would feel fatigued and some other unpleasant stuff.

Then Tessie, the receptionist, introduced me to Todd Walker, the Chief Radiation Therapist. He showed me the machine that would measure me for the radiation treatments. It was HUGE!!

At my second session, Dr. Chen marked off the area on my body where I would receive the treatments.

Then Todd and Kelly (the Radiation Therapist who would be treating me) put me on that machine and measured and marked me for treatments. Everything was totally painless! Another blessing!!

My radiation treatments will start on Monday, September 26. They will last for 20 minutes—Monday through Friday, for seven weeks. I can expect the treated area to tan (I'm already a caramel brown complexion), but not burn. Like any other tan, it will fade, and I'll get my color back. Yaaay!!

On Friday, September 23, Pap went with me to get a whole-body PET scan. I wanted to get this done BEFORE I started radiation. No rhyme or reason to it—just a personal preference. As some of my family and close friends would say, "It's a 'Joyce thing.'"

Joe, the technician, came into the prep room and injected me (didn't hurt a bit!) with a small amount of radioactive material (called a "tracer") and dye. Then, I had to wait for about 45 minutes while this stuff coursed its way through my body. I didn't feel a thing—just normal.

Then, it was time for me to meet the machine.

I am absolutely amazed at the ingenuity of the human mind to design and build these machines! The PET scan machine looks like a really big tunnel. The technician had me lie on this narrow table and insert my arms into a "sleeve-like" muff—there is no place to rest your arms. The muff was very comfortable.

I had to lie perfectly still while the technician slowly guided me through the tunnel as the machine did its scanning—in sections. He would move me a little, then stop, and the machine would make this sound (not loud), and the scanning lights would flash (not bright); then, on to the next section.

The whole process took about 30 minutes. PET scan done. I have an appointment with Dr. Mac on October 11. It may be sooner, if I can get it rescheduled.

On Monday, September 26, I had my first radiation session. Another amazing machine!

My radiation therapists, Kelly and Cat, had me lie on this narrow table—yep, another narrow table! But, this time, they took my arms and positioned them in these stirrup-looking gadgets. Very comfortable. They moved my body around, in little increments, calling off coordinates, until I was perfectly positioned.

And, someone was smart enough to have a flat-screen television mounted on the ceiling—right in the patient's line of vision. It was tuned to the local news. I'm a news/politics/current affairs addict, so—perfecto!

The machine looks like a big circle that can rotate over your body (at breast level) from left to right, or vice versa. There's a little "window" (approximately 2" x 3") in the center that changed size, depending on the movement of the "rods" in the window. I watched it make changes and heard it issue the radiation. You don't see the radiation; you just hear it. Much like getting a dental x-ray. No pain at all— except for the three "tattoos" that Kelly gave me—one on my right side, one on my left side, and one between my breasts. They each felt like a single pin prick. She and Cat will use them as guide markers.

Starting the next week, I will see Dr. Chen every Wednesday.

The radiation session lasted for 20 minutes. I now have two sessions down, 33 more to go. I have a written schedule, and I'm crossing them off as I complete them.

I believe in signs—especially GOOD signs. Guess when my last session is scheduled for? Get ready for this. It blew my mind! My last radiation session is scheduled for Friday, 11/11/11!! Wow!! And I asked if I could make my appointment for 11 a.m. My request was granted!

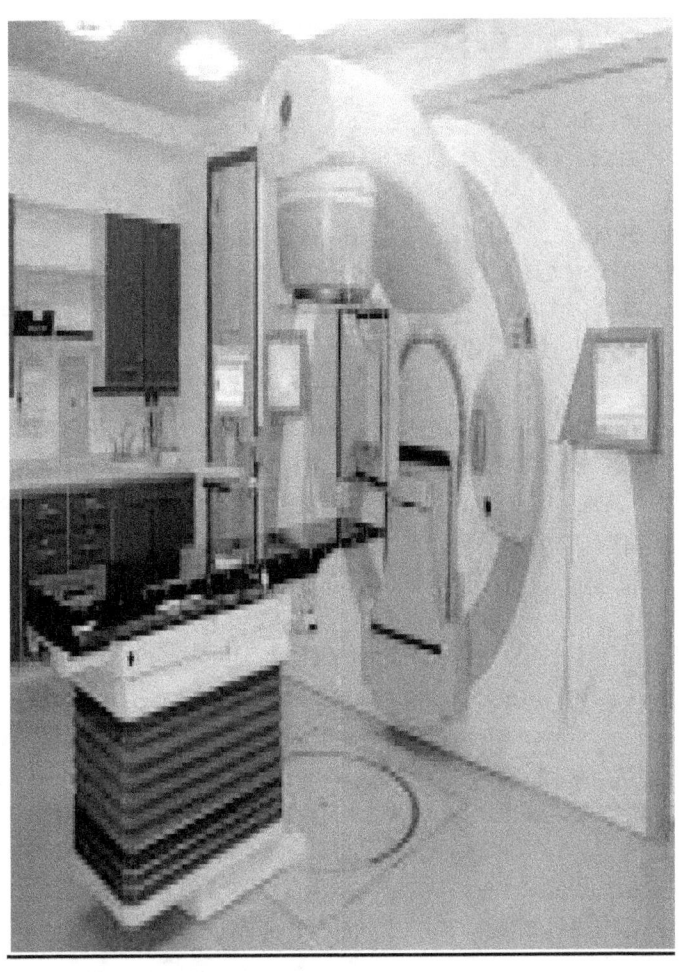

Radiation machine.

Source: breastcancerinfoblog.com

PET SCAN RESULTS

On Thursday, October 13, and I got the results of the PET scan.

When Dr. McNamara walked into the exam room, the first thing he said was, "Your PET scan was normal." It did not detect cancer in any other part of my body!

I was absolutely thrilled!! I told him that I might not hear anything else he said to me during that visit because I was so excited about the PET scan results. We both laughed, but I really did hear the rest of what he said.

He told me that I would start medication AFTER I finish radiation. My last radiation treatment is on (you may remember). . .**11/11/11 at 11 a.m.**! Because some of the medications have the potential to thin your bones, he wants me to schedule a bone density test, which I'll have done in the next week or so. That will help us to decide which medication is best for me.

I read that Vitamin D is good for fighting cancer. Dr. Mac said that research does support that statement. He ordered a blood draw to measure my Vitamin D level.

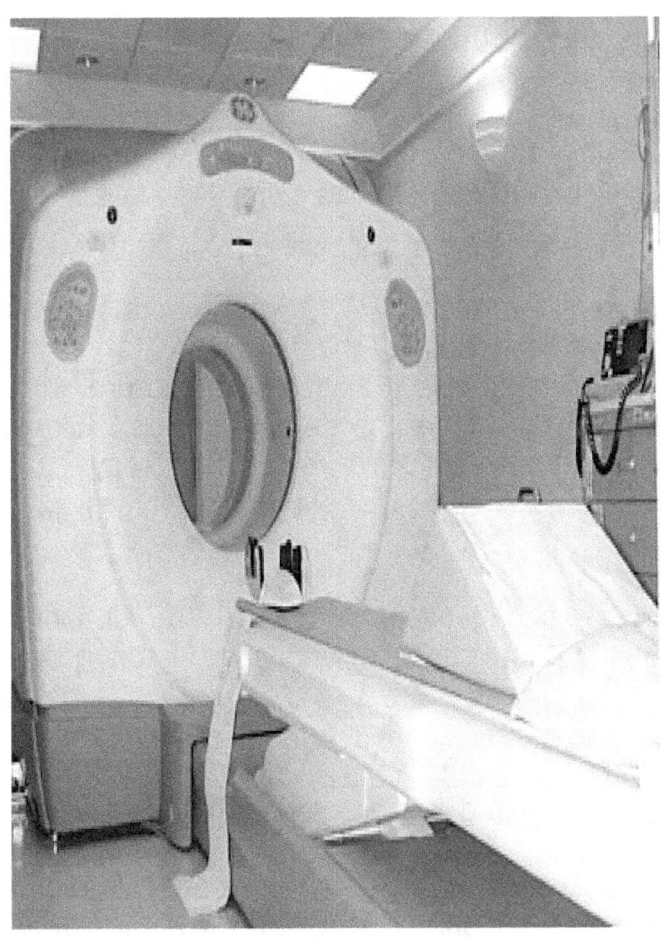

Pet scan machine.

Source: survivingcancersoon.wordpress.com

He called me the next day and told me that my level is low. It's 21. A good level is 30 and above.

So, I'll be taking 1200 IU's daily. He suggested that I get Vitamin D with calcium.

Your body makes Vitamin D when you're exposed to sunshine. The typical recommendation is 15 minutes of exposure, with 40% of your skin exposed—no sunscreen. Since I live in sunny California (it was 100° today— October 13!), I'll do that two or three times a week.

You can find many articles on the Internet about Vitamin D and cancer. Here's the link to a good one:

http://savannahnow.com/bluffton-news/2011-10-12/vitamin-d-and-breast-health

My sister-in-law, Sarah, called me and told me that her nutritionist said watercress is a good cancer fighter. Naturally, I looked it up. I'm into natural stuff! Here's the link to one of the articles:

http://www.sciencedaily.com/releases/2010/09/100914115240.htm

I am feeling really, really wonderful. My son tells people who ask him, "She acts like nothing happened." And that's the way I feel. Like nothing happened. Cancer is diabolical. It can be silent. Once the tumor was cut out of me, I was totally relieved. The silent monster (that I didn't even know was there) is gone!

The PET scan results put the cherry on top! Again, I said, "**THANK YOU, GOD!!!**"

THE WEEK OF NOVEMBER 6. WOW!!!

What a fabulous week it was! The week of November 6!!

On Tuesday, November 8, Dr. Mac told me that, after surgery (a lumpectomy) and radiation, I am cancer free!! He gave me my prescription for Tamoxifen. If I have any pre-cancerous cells in my body, the Tamoxifen will prevent them from dividing, and they will die.

I'll see Dr. Mac again on Tuesday, January 10, 2012.

On Friday, November 11 (11/11/11, at 11 a.m. [awesome!]), I had my last radiation treatment!! Oh, happy day!! And I never experienced fatigue or any of the other negative stuff I was warned about. I was my normal, energetic self throughout the entire treatment!

It was bittersweet because, over the seven-week course of radiation therapy, I developed a wonderful relationship with the Radiation Oncology staff at the South Pasadena Cancer Center: Tessie, the Receptionist; Todd, the Radiation Therapy Chief; Lara, the Registered Nurse; and my two fantastic Radiation Therapists, who administered the treatment every day for six weeks, Kelly and Cat; and then, there's Dr. Helen Chen, my Radiation Oncologist. Dr. Chen is THE BEST. Perky, positive, professional, and she really knows her stuff!

I'll see them all again on Wednesday, December 14, for my one-month, follow-up visit with Dr. Chen.

Now, back to my normal life—a life without radiation therapy!

It's important to have the love and support of your mate as you make this journey. I am blessed because Pap is giving me both, as he stands beside me and behind me! It would be a whole lot harder—on many levels—without him. I'm very thankful!

****

And I want to acknowledge the outstanding care that has been provided to me by my care givers, starting with my Primary Care Provider, Dr. Stanley Tu; Dr. Jon Foran from the Huntington-Hill Breast Center; Dr. Dawn Hills (my surgeon), Director, Surgical Breast Oncology at the City of Hope Medical Group; Dr. Helen Chen (my Radiologist); Dr. Mark McNamara (my Medical Oncologist). All of them are located in Pasadena, California.

TAMOXIFEN AND ME

I took Tamoxifen for four months--twice a day, every day.

Monday, April 2, 2012, I called my nephew, Charlie, to sing "Happy Birthday," as I do with many of my relatives. Later that day, Steve, the handyman, was in our unit repairing the bathroom faucet. We were having a casual conversation when I noticed that my words were coming out really weird. I remarked to Steve that I was having a "brain fart." He responded that it happens to all of us. When he left, I went on with my usual routine: cooking, housework, being on the computer.

When Pap came home late from work, I was busy on the computer. We had minimal conversation. He later told me that he thought I was angry with him, so he was giving me my space.

Then, on Tuesday, April 3, 2012, when it came time to get Pap up for work, I could not voice the words, "Time to get up." My mind was working. I knew that I had to tell him to get up, but I could not say the words. I did not feel strange at all. I felt fine. Finally, I was able to force the words out. Pap got up. Then I went back to sleep.

The following sequence of events is a testament to the fact that God truly does work in mysterious ways.

Shortly after I got up, my brother, Cordell, called me. Whatever he would say, I would respond with, "Um. . .um. . .um." He called our sister, Nita, and asked her if she had spoken with me that day and told her that something was wrong.

Now Pap seldom came home for lunch, but that day he did. A **few minutes(!)** after he got home, Nita called me. I was still doing the "Um" thing. I don't remember telling her that Pap was home, but she told me to give the phone to Pap. She recited the symptoms of a stroke to him, and he tested me. The two of them decided that it was time to take me to the emergency room. I felt fine, but willingly went because I knew that something wasn't right.

When we got to the emergency room, Pap explained what was happening, and they immediately seated me and started asking me questions. When the nurse asked me when I noticed that something was wrong, I told her about the "brain farts" the day before. She looked at me as if to say, "*Yesterday! And you're just now coming in?!*" She didn't understand that I was feeling fine and normal throughout this ordeal. I was admitted on the spot! They gave me an MRI, a chest x-ray, and other **totally painless** tests.

They kept me for three days. Pap stayed with me the whole time!

On the second day, Dr. Tu came to see me. He told me that I had had a mini-stroke that affected my speech center. He tested my coordination and strength. I passed with flying colors--except for my speech. I was still babbling! I couldn't get my thoughts to coordinate with my words! He arranged for a speech therapist to come to my house. (I think it was two or three times a week for six weeks.)

About a week later, the speech therapist appeared. He was a huge man (about 6' 6"). I don't remember his name, but the sessions consisted of showing me pictures of famous people and I had to say something about who they were and/or what they did.

On about the fourth session, he told me that I was doing so well that he didn't think there was anything else he could do for me. So, he ended the sessions.

My college English professor, Dr. Carol Carpenter, with whom I have stayed in contact for more than 40 years explained how the stroke had affected my speech this way: She told me that before I had the stroke, on a scale from one to ten, I was at a 12 in English fluency. Since I had the stroke, I was at a 10--still waaaaaay above average. That made me feel good and much more confident! Even now, as I talk with people, they say that they cannot tell that I had a stroke. Very blessed!

NO TAMOXIFEN AND ME!

About two weeks after I was discharged from the hospital, I went to see Dr. Mac. I told him that I had I stroke. One possible side effect of Tamoxifen is stroke. He took me off of it immediately. (I had already stopped taking it!)

About 30 years ago, I bought a book called, "Back to Eden" by Jethro Kloss. Written in the 1920s and 1930s, this book helped to create today's natural foods industry. Jethro Kloss said, "God has provided a remedy for every disease that might afflict us." I believe that.

I do not trust prescription medications because they have so many very negative--and sometimes deadly--side effects. I think I have good reasons!! Watch television long enough and a commercial will come on about some pill that will fix whatever. But when you listen to the possible side effects (they don't even list **everything**), it makes one wonder if people aren't better off with the ailment!

Since I stopped taking the Tamoxifen, I am not on ANY prescription medication and never have been.

NOTE: If your doctor **does** prescribe Tamoxifen for you, please take it--like I did. As I said, I know at least two women who took it with no problems. It may be the same for you!

FOLLOW-UP ULTRASOUNDS

In 2012, I had my first post-surgery ultrasound. The results were excellent!

In March 2013, I had another ultrasound, with the same results.

In March 2014, I had my third one. There was no change from the second one!! The doctor said after two years with no change, they now consider me to be "stable." Again, I said, **"Thank you, God!!"**

Joy!! Joy!! Joy!!

I was always joyful (after all, my name is **Joy**ce), but now I'm at a place of **GREATER** joy--like the title of this book says!

IF YOU ARE DIAGNOSED WITH STAGE 2 <u>INVASIVE DUCTAL CARCINOMA. . .</u>

Now, I am not a health care professional, but this is what I advise:

1. You can't panic! You can't freak out! It is what it is. You can't change it by panicking; you can't change it by freaking out. That will only make matters worse: high blood pressure; anxiety and panic attacks, etc.
2. Pray. And learn to calm yourself through meditation.
3. Become an active partner in your treatment. Read books. Subscribe to health newsletters. Do searches on the Internet. It's YOUR health, and it's YOUR life! Fight for it!
4. If you're not already doing it, change to a nearly all-organic diet. Conventional produce is sprayed with pesticides and herbicides. They are toxins (poisins).
5. Increase your intake of organic fresh, raw broccoli, spinach, cauliflower, watermelon. Do your own research on what foods have the highest alkalinity. Based on current

research, cancer cells cannot thrive in an alkaline body.

6. Avoid artificial sweeteners; e.g., aspartame, high fructose corn syrup, etc., because they are artificial and foreign to the body.

7. Increase your intake of water. Try to get at least eight (8) glasses per day. Do your own research on MSM powder and, if you agree with it, add it to your drinking water. Ask your doctor about it.

8. Have your Vitamin D level checked. Do your own research and consult with your doctor.

9. If you're overweight, lose those extra pounds. Don't diet (bad word!)--just change your eating habits!

10. Exercise regularly. It's good for your health. Doctors always ask if you're getting regular exercise.

11. Read labels. If you can't pronounce it, don't eat it or use it on your body.

12. Don't use deodorants that contain aluminum or parabens. According to the *World English Dictionary*, a paraben is "any ester of parahydroxybenzoic acid, some of which are used in cosmetics and pharmaceuticals and have been found in breast cancer tumours."

13. Organic, unrefined coconut oil can be used as an effective deodorant, as well as a total-body oil. That's what I use.

14. You may be iodine deficient. Organic kelp is an excellent source of iodine, but do your own research and consult with your doctor.

15. Get at least eight hours of sleep every night. Your body works on healing itself while you sleep/rest.

MY DAILY HEALTH MAINTENANCE ROUTINE

Every morning, I have my "green drink," which consists of (everything is organic):

1 cup carrot juice
Handful of spinach
2-3 spears of broccoli
1/2 heaping tsp of turmeric
1/8 tsp of kelp granules (excellent source of iodine)
1 scoop of wheat grass powder
1 clove of garlic

I put all of this in the blender for several minutes, then drink it while I take my vitamins and minerals (all vegetable capsules or gel caps--mostly 1000 mg):

Flax seed oil
Cod liver oil
Vitamin C
Calcium/Magnesium/Zinc
Grape Seed Extract Capsule
Vitamin D3
Red Yeast Rice (to control cholesterol)

I mix liquid ginger, dandelion, and cayenne extracts in a half cup of alkaline water (look up the benefits of alkaline water) and take that separately, immediately after my "green drink."

I make my own alkaline water by mixing 1/2 tsp of baking soda to a quart of water, to which I have added one tsp MSM powder (look up the benefits of MSM powder). I drink alkaline water throughout the day.

And every night (with alkaline water) I take:

Flax seed oil
Cod liver oil
Vitamin C
Calcium/Magnesium/Zinc
Grape Seed Extract Capsule
Red Yeast Rice
Low-dose aspirin (because of the stroke)
Liquid ginger, dandelion, and cayenne extracts

NOTE: I split the dosage. If the directions say "take two a day," I take one in the morning and one at night.

I snack on a mixture of (all organic) raw almonds, brazil nuts, and raisins.
I subscribe to several health newsletters and am constantly reading about maintaining good health. I also post healthful information on social media.

My diet consists of about 95% organic foods. I eat an organic, raw salad virtually every day, and have drastically reduced my consumption of refined, white sugar (I don't even buy it anymore), using organic, raw sugar instead. I read somewhere that, "if you think eating organic is expensive, try pricing cancer!" Amen!! I'm a witness!!

You must find your own course and what works best for you. I have shared what I do for those who may want to know. (I do cheat every once in a while. I'll have a scoop of ice cream, or a slice of cake, or a few potato chips. But I don't pig out, like I used to do!)

I am much more aware of my many blessings and tell God daily how grateful I am for my health and happiness.

So, if you do get a breast cancer diagnosis, don't be scared. Be grateful (it could be worse). Be positive. And pray!

I have described the procedures that I had to go through to help calm any fear you may have and to unlock a lot of the mysteries associated with a breast cancer diagnosis. **All of it was virtually painless!!**

If I can do it, so can YOU!!

Special thanks to my four doctors (Drs. Tu, Hills, McNamara, and Chen) for their support during this journey and for their enthusiastic willingness to write a foreword for this book!

Peace and love,

Joyce

See the next page for a list of my other books.

MY OTHER BOOKS

Non-Fiction
- *Line of Serenity*
- *Mother's Dozen: An Easy Recipe for Raising GREAT Kids!*
- *Madre Docena (Mother's Dozen in Spanish)*
- *THE VISION: Telling Kids That They Can Make the World a Better Place*
- *The Best Way to Keep a Man is to Let Him Go (among other things)*
- *Dear Bully: A Collection of Poems about Bullying*
- *My Simple Quotes to Live By*

Children's Fiction
- *Jette Black and Her Seven Friends*

You can read all of the books' descriptions and order them at www.goodshortbooks.com.

SPEAKING ENGAGEMENTS
I am also available for speaking engagements (television, radio, conferences, Webinars, teleseminars).

Contact me at goodshortbooks@yahoo.com.